Auriculotherapy

A Practical Guide to Ear Acupuncture

Discover Effective Techniques for Pain Relief and Healing Through Ear Acupuncture

Graham Julian Oliver

Disclaimer

The information provided in "Auriculotherapy: A Practical Guide to Ear Acupuncture" is intended for educational and informational purposes only. It is not a substitute for professional medical advice, diagnosis, or treatment. Always seek the advice of your physician or other qualified health provider with any questions you may have regarding a medical condition or treatment.

The author and publisher of this book do not endorse any specific individual, product, website, organization, or other names mentioned within. All references made in this book are for informational purposes only and do not imply any form of endorsement or recommendation.

By using this book, you acknowledge that you are solely responsible for your own health decisions and that the author and publisher shall not be liable for any damages or negative consequences arising from the use or reliance on any information provided in this book.

About This Book

Auriculotherapy: A Practical Guide to Ear Acupuncture is an invaluable resource for both beginners and seasoned practitioners looking to explore the profound healing potential of ear acupuncture. The book is structured in a way that simplifies complex techniques, offering a step-by-step approach to ensure that even those new to the field can navigate their way toward mastering auriculotherapy. Through this guide, readers will be introduced to the anatomy of the ear, the principles of reflexology, and how these ear points can influence overall body health. Furthermore, the book covers essential tools and techniques, all while addressing common concerns, providing FAQs, and outlining safety procedures.

Understanding Auriculotherapy is the first crucial step for anyone new to this healing practice. Auriculotherapy, rooted in traditional acupuncture, focuses on stimulating specific points on the ear to alleviate pain, balance bodily functions, and enhance overall wellness. The concept of reflexology underpins this approach, where the ear is seen as a microcosm of the body, with points corresponding to various organs and systems. Understanding how these points affect the body's health is essential for practitioners and patients alike. This book gives a thorough explanation of these connections, ensuring the reader grasps the fundamentals of auriculotherapy before diving deeper into practical applications.

Basic Anatomy of the Ear in Auriculotherapy provides readers with a detailed guide to the ear's structure, pinpointing the key anatomical landmarks used in treatment. It explains how specific points on the ear correlate with body parts and outlines how the nervous system interacts with these acupuncture points. Knowing how to accurately locate these points is crucial for effective treatments, and this book simplifies the process through clear, illustrative explanations. Tools and equipment, such as needles, ear seeds, and electrical stimulation devices, are introduced in a way that makes them accessible to beginners, setting the stage for confident and successful practice.

This guide then seamlessly transitions into more detailed topics, explaining the **History and Foundations of Auriculotherapy**. It delves into the origins of the practice in both China and France, highlighting key figures like Dr. Paul Nogier, who pioneered its development. The book also addresses how ear acupuncture has evolved and gained recognition globally, supported by scientific research. Auriculotherapy's role in modern integrative medicine is explored, along with common misconceptions, ethical considerations, and how tools have been refined over time to make treatments more effective.

Moving forward, the book provides practical insights into the **Tools and Techniques in Auriculotherapy**, offering an overview of different types of needles and non-invasive tools like acupressure seeds and magnets. Readers will learn how to properly locate ear points, safely insert needles, and apply ear seeds for prolonged stimulation. Advanced techniques, such as electrical stimulation and laser therapy, are introduced, making this book a comprehensive resource for those wanting to explore more sophisticated methods.

A pivotal chapter is **Identifying and Mapping Key Ear Points**, which helps readers navigate the intricate landscape of the ear's acupuncture points. This section details the three primary zones of the ear and the points corresponding to various body systems, such as the spine, digestive system, and internal organs. Special attention is given to points for treating pain, emotional well-being, and common ailments like headaches, respiratory issues, and insomnia. Mapping these points correctly is critical for treatment success, and the guide provides a clear, user-friendly approach.

For beginners, the chapter on **Step-by-Step Procedures for Beginners** breaks down the process of auriculotherapy into manageable steps. It covers setting up a treatment space, preparing the ear, and inserting needles or applying ear seeds with precision. Tips for avoiding common mistakes, understanding patient responses, and ensuring proper aftercare are also included, making it easier for new practitioners to feel confident in their practice. Additionally, the guide outlines the frequency of treatments for different conditions and how to combine auriculotherapy with other healing methods.

The book also emphasizes treating specific conditions in **Treating Common Ailments with Auriculotherapy**. This chapter provides targeted treatments for a variety of ailments, including back pain, headaches, digestive issues, menstrual cramps, and emotional disorders like stress and anxiety. Practical tips on how to stimulate points for pain relief, hormone regulation, improved sleep, and energy boosts are covered. By following the procedures outlined, readers will be able to address common health concerns through auriculotherapy with minimal difficulty.

In the section on **Safety and Contraindications in Auriculotherapy**, the book highlights the importance of patient safety, listing contraindications for specific populations, such as pregnant women, children, or individuals with pacemakers. Proper sterilization practices, needle disposal, and infection prevention are explained in detail. The guide also addresses how to handle potential allergic reactions, infections, or skin irritations that may arise during treatment, ensuring that readers are well-prepared to practice safely and effectively.

One of the most engaging aspects of this book is the integration of auriculotherapy with other healing modalities. In **Combining Auriculotherapy with Other Therapies**, the guide explains how to incorporate ear acupuncture with body acupuncture, herbal medicine, chiropractic care, and even massage therapy. The potential to enhance treatment outcomes through multi-therapy approaches is explored, and readers are provided with practical advice on using essential oils, diet changes, and mindfulness techniques alongside auriculotherapy.

Finally, **Common Concerns and FAQs in Auriculotherapy** addresses the most frequently asked questions by both practitioners and patients. It offers clear answers on the safety, effectiveness, and duration of treatments, while also providing guidance on self-administration, combining auriculotherapy with other treatments, and managing any side effects that may occur post-session. This section is especially valuable for those new to the practice, offering reassurance and practical advice to overcome any hesitations.

Table of Contents

Introduction Headings

Definition of Auriculotherapy and Its Origins

Auriculotherapy, or ear acupuncture, is a technique involving the stimulation of points on the outer ear to treat various physical and emotional health issues. Originating from ancient Chinese practices and developed further in France by Dr. Paul Nogier in the 1950s, it is based on the idea that the ear represents a micro system of the entire body, where each point corresponds to a specific area or function. Practitioners use needles, laser, or even pressure techniques to activate these points and stimulate the body's self-healing mechanisms.

In practical application, auriculotherapy involves identifying points on the ear that connect to health concerns, from pain management to mental wellness. For beginners, it's essential to understand the ear's map, which indicates the corresponding body parts. Simple stimulation methods, such as applying pressure to specific ear points, can be done at home using clean hands or a tool, while more complex techniques, like needle insertion, should be administered by a trained professional.

How Auriculotherapy Connects to Traditional Acupuncture

Auriculotherapy aligns closely with traditional acupuncture, sharing the principle that the body can be influenced through stimulating certain points to restore balance. However, while traditional acupuncture involves the entire body, auriculotherapy focuses solely on the ear, offering a more targeted, accessible method. Both practices aim to harmonize Qi (life energy), relieve pain, and promote healing, but auriculotherapy is often a suitable alternative for those who prefer non-invasive techniques or are new to acupuncture.

When performing auriculotherapy, practitioners use points on the ear that correspond to the body's meridian channels, similar to traditional acupuncture but condensed within the ear's micro system. For at-home practice, beginners might start with gentle ear massage techniques on stress-related points, such as the Shen Men point, known for its calming effects. Advanced auriculotherapy, often conducted in clinics, uses specialized needles or lasers to activate deeper responses.

Key Benefits of Auriculotherapy for Pain Relief and Healing

Auriculotherapy is widely recognized for its benefits in pain relief, helping conditions like back pain, migraines, and arthritis. By stimulating specific ear points, the practice can activate the body's endorphin release, providing natural pain relief and improving one's overall sense of well-being. Beyond pain management, auriculotherapy can help with mental health issues like anxiety, insomnia, and even addictive cravings, providing a holistic approach to health.

In practice, auriculotherapy is a flexible technique that can be integrated into a broader wellness routine. For pain relief, beginners can try pressing on the ear's sympathetic point, located in the upper section, to reduce tension and promote relaxation. With regular application, these techniques can create cumulative effects, making auriculotherapy a valuable tool in both acute and chronic pain management.

The Concept of Reflexology in Ear Acupuncture

Reflexology in auriculotherapy involves mapping out areas on the ear that correspond to specific organs and systems in the body. This concept builds on the idea that the ear is a micro system reflecting the entire body, allowing practitioners to stimulate reflex points on the ear to relieve issues elsewhere. Each point on the ear, from the lobe to the upper rim, represents a different body part, much like foot reflexology.

For practical use, reflexology requires a basic understanding of the ear's map. Beginners might start by identifying key reflex points, such as the stomach or spine, on the ear chart and practicing gentle massage or acupressure on these spots. With practice, users can learn to address specific issues, using reflexology on the ear to support the health of the corresponding body part.

The Role of the Ear in Influencing Various Body Functions

The ear has a profound connection with the body's nervous and circulatory systems, influencing several body functions through its rich network of nerve endings and blood vessels. In auriculotherapy, stimulating certain points on the ear can activate the body's parasympathetic nervous system, leading to relaxation and improved bodily functions such as digestion, heart rate, and hormonal balance.

To engage these functions, beginners can apply light pressure on the vagus nerve area, found near the concha, or the hollow part of the ear. This can help calm the body and improve digestion, making it a practical point for stress relief and managing digestive issues. By focusing on these points regularly, users can encourage healthier bodily functions and improve their resilience against stress.

Definition of auriculotherapy and its origins

How Auriculotherapy Connects to Traditional Acupuncture

Auriculotherapy, or ear acupuncture, is rooted in the principles of traditional acupuncture but focuses specifically on the ear as a micro system reflecting the entire body. In traditional acupuncture, fine needles are inserted into various points on the body's meridians to stimulate energy flow or "Qi." Auriculotherapy operates similarly, but by targeting specific points on the ear, it influences other parts of the body, as each section of the ear corresponds to different organs and systems. This connection aligns auriculotherapy with traditional Chinese medicine by supporting the balance of energy throughout the body.

Practitioners begin by identifying specific ear points that relate to areas needing relief. For example, by placing a needle in the "liver" point on the ear, the practitioner aims to improve liver function and alleviate related symptoms, such as stress or digestive issues. Using methods like electro stimulation or small acupressure beads, auriculotherapy offers a practical approach to targeting health concerns, drawing from acupuncture's foundational theory while providing a more localized, focused technique.

Key Benefits of Auriculotherapy for Pain Relief and Healing

Auriculotherapy offers a range of benefits, particularly for pain management, stress relief, and overall wellness. By stimulating specific points on the ear, practitioners can provide targeted pain relief, making it useful for conditions like migraines, chronic pain, and even post-surgical discomfort. As an adjunct to traditional medicine, auriculotherapy can enhance the effects of conventional treatments, helping to relax the nervous system and reduce inflammation naturally.

Beyond pain relief, auriculotherapy also aids in healing processes and improves emotional well-being. The technique has been shown to reduce anxiety, alleviate insomnia, and help with addictions by targeting points linked to emotional centers. With consistent treatments, patients often report feeling more balanced and in control of their symptoms, as the therapy promotes holistic healing by gently realigning bodily functions.

The Concept of Reflexology in Ear Acupuncture

In auriculotherapy, the principle of reflexology suggests that each part of the ear reflects the whole body, with various points on the ear corresponding to specific organs or systems. By stimulating these points, practitioners can impact distant body areas. For example, the lobe of the ear represents the head and face, while areas on the upper ear relate to internal organs. This mirror effect allows practitioners to address health issues across the body by working solely on the ear.

The process involves locating the correct points, often with the help of diagrams or palpation, where the ear may feel tender or warm, indicating an underlying issue. Practitioners apply pressure, needles, or even seeds to stimulate these reflex points. This form of reflexology makes auriculotherapy an effective tool for addressing internal health concerns through external stimulation, simplifying the process for patients who may not be comfortable with full-body acupuncture.

The Role of the Ear in Influencing Various Body Functions

The ear's rich network of nerves makes it uniquely influential in regulating body functions, as it connects to the vagus nerve, which controls numerous bodily processes, including digestion, heart rate, and immune response. Through auriculotherapy, stimulating these nerve-connected points on the ear can enhance various physiological functions. By influencing nerve pathways directly from the ear, practitioners can encourage relaxation, improve blood flow, and help reduce pain.

To apply this, practitioners focus on points tied to specific systems; for instance, stimulating the "kidney" point can support renal health, while the "lung" point may help with respiratory issues. This systematic approach leverages the ear's connection to both the nervous and circulatory systems, enabling auriculotherapy to support the body's natural healing by tapping into its neurophysiologic pathways.

Basic Anatomy of the Ear in Auriculotherapy

Main Anatomical Landmarks of the Ear Used in Treatment

In auriculotherapy, key anatomical landmarks on the ear provide foundational reference points to locate acupuncture areas. These landmarks include the helix, antihelix, tragus, antitragus, and lobe. Each of these areas connects to specific body parts, with the lobe often corresponding to the head and the upper parts of the ear relating to lower body regions. Beginners can use visual charts to familiarize themselves with these areas for accurate point location during treatment.

The auricle, or outer ear, serves as a microcosm of the body, meaning each part of the ear represents a different bodily region. The ear is mapped similarly to an upside-down fetus, with the head represented at the earlobe and the lower limbs at the top of the ear. Knowing these landmarks allows for targeted treatment, whether addressing pain, stress, or other symptoms. Consistent practice with anatomical charts will help beginners identify points accurately over time.

Specific Ear Points Related to Various Body Parts

Auriculotherapy utilizes specific ear points to target body parts for pain relief and therapeutic effects. For example, the Shen Men point, located on the upper part of the antihelix, is often used to reduce stress and promote relaxation. Similarly, the lung point, located within the concha, can be beneficial for respiratory issues. Identifying and understanding these points allow practitioners to tailor treatments to specific ailments.

For beginners, it's essential to have a clear understanding of the ear map, which demonstrates the body's organs and regions on the ear. Using an ear acupuncture chart, one can precisely locate these points and apply gentle pressure or needles as appropriate. Consistent practice on a model ear can help beginners quickly identify points and develop confidence in targeting the correct regions.

How the Nervous System Interacts with Ear Acupuncture Points

Auriculotherapy works by stimulating specific ear points that communicate with the brain and nervous system. When these points are pressed or needled, they send signals through cranial and spinal nerves, which relay messages to various organs or body parts. This process can reduce pain, alleviate stress, and improve organ function, as the brain adjusts responses to these signals.

The ear is uniquely sensitive due to its rich nerve supply, making it an ideal area for therapeutic stimulation. By understanding how auriculotherapy affects the nervous system, practitioners can select points that offer direct relief for specific conditions, such as using the Shen Men point for calming effects. Through repeated application, these techniques can provide both physical and mental health benefits, effectively harnessing the nervous system's natural responses.

Importance of Proper Ear Point Location for Effective Results

Accurate ear point location is essential in auriculotherapy to achieve desired therapeutic outcomes. Each ear point connects with specific body parts, and even a slight misplacement can lead to ineffective treatment. Using visual aids, such as ear maps and acupuncture charts, can help beginners learn the precise positioning of each point.

Effective auriculotherapy relies on consistent practice in locating these points with precision. Many practitioners start with non-invasive methods, such as using ear seeds or gentle pressure, before progressing to needles. Ensuring the correct point placement helps maximize the treatment's benefits, whether targeting pain, digestion, or mental wellness, and builds the practitioner's skill in providing targeted, reliable relief.

Overview of Tools and Equipment Used in Auriculotherapy

Auriculotherapy requires specific tools to accurately stimulate points on the ear. Basic tools include ear seeds, tiny beads placed on adhesive tape for non-invasive point pressure, and acupuncture needles for more advanced treatments. Practitioners may also use a point detector, a handheld device that helps locate active points on the ear by sensing electrical resistance changes, which can guide beginners in precise targeting.

Ear acupressure kits often include tweezers for placing seeds and sterilizing swabs to maintain cleanliness. For those practicing at home, a beginner-friendly option is to start with ear seeds, which can be pressed to stimulate points without needles. Familiarizing oneself with these tools provides a more accessible introduction to auriculotherapy, offering hands-on experience with minimal discomfort or risk.

CHAPTER 1:

History and Foundations of Auriculotherapy

Origin and Evolution of Auriculotherapy in China and France

Auriculotherapy traces its roots to ancient Chinese medicine, where the ear was recognized as a microcosm of the body, reflecting various bodily functions and conditions. Early Chinese practitioners utilized ear points to diagnose and treat ailments. In the mid-20th century, this practice gained prominence in France through the work of Dr. Paul Nogier, who expanded its application and introduced a systematic mapping of ear points, leading to the evolution of modern auriculotherapy techniques.

In France, Nogier's research integrated traditional Chinese concepts with Western medical practices, establishing auriculotherapy as a legitimate therapeutic modality. His innovative approach laid the foundation for further research and development in ear acupuncture, making it a popular treatment method in both Europe and beyond.

Pioneering Research and Development of Ear Acupuncture

The development of ear acupuncture saw significant advancements through rigorous research and clinical studies that validated its efficacy. Early trials in France explored the effectiveness of auriculotherapy for pain management, demonstrating promising results. Researchers conducted experiments involving a wide range of conditions, paving the way for ear acupuncture to be recognized as a valuable tool for holistic healing.

Additionally, ongoing research continues to refine the techniques and broaden the scope of auriculotherapy. Modern studies explore its applications in stress relief, addiction treatment, and various physical ailments, ensuring that ear acupuncture remains relevant and scientifically supported in contemporary medicine.

Key Figures in the Field, Including Dr. Paul Nogier

Dr. Paul Nogier is often considered the father of modern auriculotherapy. His pioneering work in the 1950s led to the development of ear maps that correlate specific points on the ear with various body parts and functions. Nogier's dedication to research and clinical practice transformed ear acupuncture into a structured therapeutic approach, gaining recognition among healthcare practitioners.

Other notable figures include Dr. Tchao, who contributed to the standardization of auriculotherapy practices, and numerous researchers and practitioners worldwide who have expanded on Nogier's foundation. Their collective efforts have elevated the status of ear acupuncture, fostering a growing community of practitioners committed to advancing the field.

Differences between Auriculotherapy and Traditional Acupuncture

Auriculotherapy specifically focuses on the ear, utilizing distinct points that correspond to the entire body. In contrast, traditional acupuncture targets various points across the body, often following meridian pathways. This specialization makes auriculotherapy a convenient and accessible treatment option for conditions like pain and stress, as it can be performed with minimal intervention.

Practically, auriculotherapy can be done using various techniques, including needle insertion, ear seeds, or electrical stimulation. The concentrated focus on the ear allows practitioners to address a wide array of issues efficiently, making it an attractive option for both patients and practitioners seeking non-invasive treatment methods.

Role of Auriculotherapy in Modern Integrative Medicine

In today's healthcare landscape, auriculotherapy has emerged as a complementary treatment within integrative medicine. Its effectiveness in managing pain, anxiety, and addiction has led many practitioners to incorporate ear acupuncture into holistic treatment plans. This integrative approach aligns well with the principles of treating the whole person rather than just the symptoms of a condition.

Practitioners often combine auriculotherapy with other modalities, such as nutritional counseling and stress management techniques, to enhance patient outcomes. This collaborative approach allows for a comprehensive understanding of a patient's health, addressing physical, emotional, and psychological well-being.

Global Recognition and Acceptance of Ear Acupuncture

Auriculotherapy has gained significant global acceptance, with numerous practitioners and clinics integrating it into their services. International conferences, training programs, and research publications have contributed to its growing popularity among healthcare providers and patients alike. Countries like the United States, Canada, and Australia have seen a rise in interest, reflecting a shift towards more holistic healthcare approaches.

The recognition of auriculotherapy by various medical associations further legitimizes its practice. Training programs and certifications for practitioners are becoming more widespread, allowing for standardized methods and increased accessibility to this effective treatment.

Scientific Basis and Research Support for Auriculotherapy

Research supports auriculotherapy effectiveness, particularly in pain relief and management. Clinical studies have demonstrated that stimulating specific ear points can trigger physiological responses, such as the release of endorphins and changes in neurotransmitter levels, leading to improved outcomes for patients. This scientific backing is essential for integrating auriculotherapy into conventional medical practices.

Ongoing research continues to explore the mechanisms of action behind ear acupuncture, providing further evidence of its therapeutic benefits. As more studies validate its efficacy, auriculotherapy is increasingly viewed as a credible and effective treatment option in pain management and other health concerns.

How Auriculotherapy Relates to Holistic Healing Principles

Auriculotherapy embodies the principles of holistic healing by recognizing the interconnectedness of the body and mind. By treating the ear as a microcosm of the entire body, practitioners can address physical symptoms while considering emotional and psychological factors. This holistic perspective fosters a deeper understanding of patients' health, encouraging treatments that resonate with their overall well-being.

Practically, auriculotherapy sessions often begin with a thorough assessment of the patient's physical and emotional state. By tailoring treatments to individual needs, practitioners can effectively promote healing on multiple levels, enhancing the overall effectiveness of the therapy.

Common Misconceptions and Myths about Ear Acupuncture

Many misconceptions surround auriculotherapy, with some believing it to be a painful or unsafe procedure. However, ear acupuncture is generally well-tolerated, and practitioners use various methods, such as ear seeds, to minimize discomfort. Educating patients about the gentle nature of the practice can help alleviate concerns and encourage them to explore its benefits.

Another common myth is that auriculotherapy is only effective for specific conditions. In reality, ear acupuncture has a broad range of applications, from pain relief to anxiety management and even addiction treatment. Understanding the versatility of auriculotherapy can empower patients to consider it as a viable option for various health challenges.

How Ear Acupuncture Maps Were Developed and Refined

The development of ear acupuncture maps was a critical advancement in auriculotherapy, providing a visual representation of points corresponding to various body parts. Dr. Paul Nogier's initial mapping was based on his clinical observations and empirical research, leading to the identification of specific points linked to different physical and emotional conditions.

Since then, these maps have been refined through ongoing research and feedback from practitioners. Updated maps incorporate findings from clinical studies, ensuring that they remain relevant and effective for modern practice. This ongoing refinement enhances the precision and efficacy of auriculotherapy treatments.

Evolution of Tools Used in Ear Acupuncture Treatments

The tools used in auriculotherapy have evolved significantly, adapting to modern medical practices and patient needs. Initially, practitioners primarily used needles for stimulation; however, advancements have introduced alternatives such as ear seeds, electrical stimulators, and laser therapy. These tools provide flexibility in treatment options, accommodating different patient preferences and comfort levels.

Modern practitioners often select tools based on the specific condition being treated and the patient's comfort. For instance, ear seeds allow for extended stimulation over time, while electrical stimulation can enhance the intensity of treatment without discomfort. This evolution in tools makes auriculotherapy more accessible and effective for a wider range of patients.

Early Experiments and Trials in Pain Relief through Ear Acupuncture

Early experiments in auriculotherapy focused on its potential for pain relief, leading to groundbreaking findings. Clinical trials conducted in the mid-20th century demonstrated that stimulation of specific ear points could significantly reduce pain levels in patients with chronic conditions. These early successes prompted further research and interest in ear acupuncture as a valid treatment modality.

The promising results from these trials laid the groundwork for contemporary practices. As more healthcare providers began integrating auriculotherapy into pain management protocols, it gained traction as a complementary approach within the larger medical community.

Ethical Considerations in the Practice of Auriculotherapy

Ethical considerations are paramount in the practice of auriculotherapy, as practitioners must prioritize patient safety and informed consent. Ensuring that patients understand the potential benefits and limitations of treatment is crucial for maintaining trust and transparency. Practitioners should also be aware of their scope of practice and refer patients to other healthcare providers when necessary.

Additionally, the practice of auriculotherapy should be grounded in evidence-based techniques, respecting the individual needs of each patient. This commitment to ethical practice not only enhances patient outcomes but also fosters a professional environment within the growing field of auriculotherapy.

CHAPTER 2:

Tools and Techniques in Auriculotherapy

Types of Needles Used for Ear Acupuncture

In ear acupuncture, the most commonly used needles are fine, sterile, single-use acupuncture needles, typically 0.12mm to 0.20mm in diameter. These needles are designed specifically for auricular points and are generally shorter than those used for body acupuncture, usually around 5-15mm long. Understanding the appropriate needle types is crucial for minimizing discomfort and maximizing therapeutic benefits.

Additionally, there are specialized needles known as "ear tacks" or "ear pins," which are small and can be left in place for several days. These are ideal for ongoing treatments and can be combined with other therapies, such as acupressure seeds or magnets, for enhanced effects. Familiarizing yourself with these options allows practitioners to choose the most effective tools based on the patient's needs.

Using Acupressure Seeds and Magnets for Non-Invasive Treatments

Acupressure seeds, also known as "ear seeds," are small, adhesive seeds from the Vaccaria plant that can be applied to specific points on the ear. To use them, simply clean the area, apply the seed to the identified point, and press down gently to adhere. This method is non-invasive and provides a gradual, continuous stimulation to the acupuncture points, making it suitable for patients who may be apprehensive about needles.

Magnets can also be utilized in a similar fashion. They are placed on acupuncture points using adhesive patches and offer a gentle magnetic stimulation. For both seeds and magnets, they can be worn for several days, providing ongoing relief without the need for regular clinic visits. It's important to instruct patients on when and how to reapply or remove these non-invasive tools.

How to Locate Specific Acupuncture Points on the Ear

Locating acupuncture points on the ear requires a basic understanding of auricular anatomy and reference charts that depict the various points. The ear can be divided into sections that correspond to different organs and systems in the body. Using these maps, practitioners can identify points such as Shen Men, which is associated with relaxation, or the point for pain relief.

To accurately locate these points, gently palpate the ear and look for depressions or areas of tenderness. Once identified, mark the locations lightly with a washable marker or use a pencil to ensure precise needle placement. This visual and tactile approach enhances accuracy and effectiveness in treatment.

Proper Sterilization and Safety Practices

Before beginning any auriculotherapy session, it is vital to ensure that all needles and tools are sterile to prevent infections. Use a commercial autoclave for sterilizing reusable equipment, and always have single-use needles readily available for patients. Clean the treatment area with alcohol swabs or antiseptic wipes to maintain a hygienic environment.

Safety practices also include using gloves during treatment and disposing of used needles in a designated sharps container. Educating patients on post-treatment care, such as keeping the ear dry and avoiding irritation, further promotes safety and effectiveness in healing.

Best Practices for Inserting and Removing Ear Needles

When inserting ear needles, begin by holding the needle with a firm grip and gently piercing the skin at a 15-degree angle. Ensure that the needle is inserted only to the depth necessary to stimulate the point without causing undue pain. A quick, smooth motion helps minimize discomfort for the patient.

For removal, grasp the needle firmly and pull it out slowly and steadily. After removal, apply a gentle pressure to the site with a cotton ball to prevent any bleeding. Always inspect the insertion site afterward for any signs of irritation or infection, providing appropriate advice on care if needed.

Frequency and Duration of Typical Auriculotherapy Sessions

Typical auriculotherapy sessions last between 20 to 45 minutes, depending on the patient's needs and the complexity of the treatment. For pain management or specific conditions, practitioners often recommend sessions two to three times a week. This frequency helps in achieving quicker relief and better results over time.

Patients may also be encouraged to engage in at-home care with ear seeds or magnets in between professional sessions. This combination allows for continuous treatment, maximizing the effectiveness of the auriculotherapy approach and promoting faster healing.

How to Apply Ear Seeds for Prolonged Stimulation

Applying ear seeds involves selecting appropriate points based on the patient's condition, cleaning the ear, and then carefully adhering the seeds to the points. Use a pair of tweezers to pick up the seeds for better precision and to avoid contamination. Press down firmly to ensure they stick securely to the ear.

Instruct patients to apply gentle pressure to the seeds throughout the day, which can enhance the stimulation and effectiveness. This at-home technique allows for sustained treatment beyond office visits, encouraging patient engagement in their healing process.

Using Electrical Stimulation Devices for Advanced Treatments

Electrical stimulation devices, often called electro-acupuncture units, can enhance the effects of traditional needle acupuncture. These devices are connected to the needles once they are inserted, delivering a mild electrical current that stimulates the acupuncture points. Start with a low frequency and gradually increase as tolerated by the patient.

Before using electrical stimulation, ensure the patient understands the process and is comfortable with it. Monitor the patient closely during treatment for any adverse reactions, adjusting the settings as necessary to ensure a safe and effective experience.

Overview of Laser Therapy in Auriculotherapy

Laser therapy in auriculotherapy utilizes low-level lasers to stimulate acupuncture points without the need for needles. The practitioner targets specific points on the ear with a handheld laser device, providing a pain-free treatment option. This method is particularly beneficial for patients with needle phobias or those seeking a non-invasive alternative.

The treatment typically lasts about 10-20 minutes per session, and patients can expect similar results to traditional acupuncture. Practitioners should educate patients on the benefits and limitations of laser therapy, ensuring they understand how it can complement other auriculotherapy methods.

Techniques for Stimulating Points Manually Using Fingers

Manual stimulation of acupuncture points can be performed by using fingers to apply pressure directly to specific points on the ear. This technique can be particularly useful for patients who prefer not to use needles or other invasive methods. Begin by locating the appropriate point and applying firm but gentle pressure for 30 seconds to a minute.

Encourage patients to practice this technique at home as a form of self-care. Regular manual stimulation can enhance the effects of other treatments and help patients develop a deeper understanding of their own bodies and responses to therapy.

How to Use Maps and Charts to Guide Treatment

Using maps and charts is essential for effectively guiding auriculotherapy treatments. Familiarize yourself with various diagrams that indicate the specific points associated with different bodily functions or conditions. These visual aids provide a clear reference for practitioners and can be printed out for patient education.

During treatment, refer to these maps to ensure accuracy in point selection. Additionally, educating patients about these maps empowers them to understand their treatment better and promotes active participation in their healing process.

Importance of Patient Comfort and Relaxation During Sessions

Creating a comfortable and relaxing environment is crucial for effective auriculotherapy. Ensure that the treatment space is quiet, with soft lighting and calming music to help patients feel at ease. Discuss any concerns with the patient beforehand to alleviate anxiety and foster a trusting relationship.

Encouraging deep breathing or meditation techniques during the session can also enhance relaxation, allowing for a more successful treatment. When patients are relaxed, they are more likely to experience the full benefits of auriculotherapy, leading to improved outcomes.

Troubleshooting Common Issues with Needle Placement

Common issues with needle placement include improper angle, excessive depth, or placing the needle on the wrong point. To troubleshoot, always check the needle's position after insertion and make any necessary adjustments. If a patient reports discomfort or pain, carefully remove the needle and reassess the location.

Another issue may arise from the patient's anatomical differences, making certain points difficult to locate.

CHAPTER 3:

Identifying and Mapping Key Ear Points

Overview of the Three Primary Zones of the Ear

Auriculotherapy divides the ear into three main zones: the outer ear (auricle), the middle ear, and the inner ear. Each zone corresponds to specific areas of the body, allowing practitioners to target various health concerns. For instance, the outer ear is generally associated with the body's surface conditions, while the inner ear relates to internal organ functions. Understanding these zones helps in effectively diagnosing and treating health issues through ear acupuncture.

To perform an ear acupuncture session, start by visually dividing the ear into these three zones. Use a clean, well-lit space and a good quality ear chart to reference specific points. By familiarizing yourself with these zones, you can accurately select the appropriate acupuncture points to address the patient's needs, ensuring a comprehensive approach to treatment.

Key Points for Treating Pain Relief in Different Parts of the Body

For effective pain relief, it is essential to know the key acupuncture points that correspond to specific body areas. For instance, points such as the Helix and Antihelix can be stimulated to alleviate pain in the back, neck, and limbs. Using fine needles or ear seeds can help in triggering these points, promoting the release of endorphins, which are natural pain relievers.

Begin by palpating the ear to locate sensitive areas that correspond to the patient's pain. Once identified, insert needles or apply pressure to these points for 20 to 30 minutes. It's crucial to check in with the patient regularly to gauge their pain levels and adjust the treatment accordingly.

How to Identify the Shen Men Point for Calming and Stress Relief

The Shen Men point, often referred to as the "Spirit Gate," is located on the triangular fossa of the ear. It is vital for promoting relaxation and reducing stress. To locate this point, find the triangular fossa and identify the highest point within it. This area is sensitive to touch and can be stimulated through gentle acupressure or acupuncture.

To use the Shen Men point for calming effects, apply pressure for about 1-2 minutes, or insert a needle for 20 minutes. This practice can be beneficial for individuals experiencing anxiety or insomnia, helping them to achieve a state of calm and tranquility.

Points That Affect the Spine, Digestion, and Internal Organs

Specific ear acupuncture points target spinal health, digestion, and internal organ function. For instance, the Point of the Spine is located near the outer edge of the ear, while points related to the stomach and intestines can be found along the antihelix. To treat issues like back pain or digestive disturbances, these points should be stimulated.

Begin by gently palpating the ear to locate these points and assess sensitivity. After identifying the areas, apply acupressure or needles, allowing the patient to relax for 20-30 minutes. This approach helps to improve organ function and alleviate discomfort in associated body areas.

Ear Points Related to Emotional Well-Being and Mental Health

Several ear acupuncture points are specifically linked to emotional and mental health, including the point for the Heart and the point for the Liver. These points are crucial for managing feelings of stress, anxiety, and depression. To find these points, refer to a detailed ear map that outlines their specific locations.

To activate these points, apply gentle pressure or acupuncture needles for a duration of 20 minutes.

Patients often experience immediate relief from emotional distress, which can help in promoting overall mental well-being.

Mapping Points for Hormone Regulation and Metabolism

Hormone regulation and metabolism can be influenced through specific ear points, including those corresponding to the adrenal and thyroid glands. These points can help manage conditions related to hormonal imbalances. To find these points, refer to a professional auricular acupuncture chart that clearly indicates where these critical areas are located.

Once identified, apply acupressure or acupuncture needles to these points for about 20-30 minutes. This method can effectively support hormonal balance and metabolic health, helping to address issues such as fatigue, weight gain, or irregular cycles.

Locating Points for Headaches and Migraines

To alleviate headaches and migraines, it's essential to know the specific ear points that can provide relief. Key points include the Point of the Occiput and points along the helix. These points are typically sensitive in individuals experiencing headaches. To locate them, palpate the ear and identify areas of tenderness.

Once located, use acupuncture or acupressure techniques on these points for 20 minutes. Patients often report significant relief from headache symptoms, making this a practical technique for both acute and chronic conditions.

How Ear Acupuncture Points Correspond to Skeletal Systems

Understanding the correlation between ear acupuncture points and the skeletal system is crucial for treating musculoskeletal issues. For example, points on the ear can correspond to specific bones or joints in the body.

By referencing an ear map, practitioners can identify these connections effectively.

When treating skeletal issues, locate the relevant points and apply needles or pressure. This technique helps in alleviating pain and promoting healing in the corresponding skeletal areas, enhancing overall mobility and function.

Using Charts to Identify Points for Respiratory Issues

Using visual charts is essential for identifying ear acupuncture points associated with respiratory conditions. Points like the Lung point and the Bronchial point can be located along the ear's antihelix. These points are beneficial for treating asthma, allergies, and other respiratory ailments.

Once you have identified these points, apply gentle pressure or acupuncture needles. Treatments typically last around 20 minutes, offering significant relief from respiratory symptoms and improving lung function.

Reflex Points on the Ear for Boosting Immune Function

Several reflex points on the ear can help boost the immune system, including the point for the Thymus. These points are important for enhancing the body's natural defenses. To find these points, utilize an ear acupuncture chart for reference.

To stimulate the immune function, apply acupressure or acupuncture techniques on these points for about 20 minutes. This practice can strengthen immune responses, helping the body to better combat infections and illnesses.

Special Points for Managing Insomnia and Sleep Disorders

To address insomnia and sleep disorders, specific ear points like the Insomnia point and the Calm point are particularly effective. These points can be found on the ear's surface and are essential for promoting restful sleep. A detailed ear chart will guide you to these critical locations.

For treatment, apply gentle acupressure or acupuncture needles to these points for 20-30 minutes. This method can significantly improve sleep quality and help patients achieve a deeper, more restorative rest.

Points for Addressing Addiction and Behavioral Health

Ear acupuncture is an effective tool for managing addiction and behavioral health issues, with key points like the Addiction point located on the ear. These points can aid in reducing cravings and promoting emotional balance. Use an ear chart to accurately identify these crucial areas.

Once located, apply acupuncture needles or acupressure for approximately 20 minutes. This treatment can provide support for individuals dealing with addiction, enhancing their recovery journey and promoting healthier coping mechanisms.

The Importance of Precision in Ear Point Mapping

Precision in ear point mapping is essential for effective treatment outcomes. Accurate identification of ear points ensures that the correct areas are stimulated for optimal results. Practitioners should always use reliable charts and anatomical references when locating points on the ear.

To enhance precision, regularly practice palpation techniques to familiarize yourself with the ear's anatomy. This skill will help you deliver targeted treatments and improve patient satisfaction by addressing their specific health concerns effectively.

CHAPTER 4:

Step-by-Step Procedures for Beginners

Setting up a calm and hygienic treatment space

To create an effective treatment environment for auriculotherapy, begin by selecting a quiet and comfortable location. Ensure the room is free from distractions and has adequate lighting. Use a clean table or surface where the patient can comfortably recline. You may also want to include calming elements such as soft music, essential oils, or soothing colors to promote relaxation.

Hygiene is crucial in any acupuncture setting. Wash your hands thoroughly before and after each treatment, and ensure all tools and surfaces are sanitized. Prepare all necessary supplies, such as needles, cotton balls, or ear seeds, and store them in a clean, organized manner. Consider laying down a clean towel or disposable paper on the treatment surface to maintain cleanliness throughout the session.

Preparing the ear for acupuncture or acupressure

Before starting the treatment, it's important to assess the patient's ears and educate them on what to expect. Begin by cleaning the ear with an alcohol swab to reduce the risk of infection and enhance comfort. Inspect the ear for any signs of irritation, inflammation, or abnormalities that may require special attention. This initial assessment will help guide your treatment approach.

Once the ear is clean, take time to explain the acupuncture points and their intended effects to the patient. Discuss how the ear corresponds to different parts of the body, as understanding this will empower the patient during the treatment. For acupressure, gently palpate the relevant points to ensure the patient is comfortable before proceeding.

Step-by-step guide for inserting needles correctly

To insert acupuncture needles correctly, first, select the appropriate needle size based on the treatment area and patient's comfort. Hold the needle between your thumb and index finger, ensuring you have a firm grip. Position the needle at a 15 to 30-degree angle towards the selected acupuncture point, then quickly but gently insert it with a swift motion, allowing it to penetrate to the desired depth.

After insertion, observe the patient for any signs of discomfort or adverse reactions. If resistance is felt, do not force the needle; instead, gently adjust the angle or reposition it. Once the needles are correctly placed, ensure the patient is comfortable and relaxed. Explain to them that they may feel a slight tingling sensation, which indicates that the treatment is working.

How to apply ear seeds for self-treatment at home

Ear seeds are an effective and non-invasive way to perform auriculotherapy at home. Start by identifying the specific acupuncture points on the ear that correspond to your health concerns. Use a clean tweezer to pick up the ear seeds, which are small, adhesive seeds or beads often derived from the Vaccaria plant. Place a seed directly on the designated point, applying gentle pressure to ensure it adheres properly.

Once the seeds are in place, apply light pressure on them throughout the day. You can stimulate the points by gently pressing or massaging them whenever you feel discomfort or need relief. Ear seeds can remain on the ear for several days, allowing for continuous treatment. Be sure to clean the area regularly and replace any seeds that fall off or lose their adhesion.

Duration and pressure levels for effective treatments

For effective auriculotherapy treatments, the duration can vary depending on the condition being addressed. Generally, needle retention times can range from 20 to 40 minutes. During this time, ensure the patient remains relaxed and free from distractions. For ear seeds, it's recommended to stimulate them for a few minutes several times a day, depending on individual needs.

When applying pressure during treatment, it's essential to gauge the patient's comfort level. Start with light pressure and gradually increase as the patient acclimates. A good rule of thumb is to use enough pressure to feel a slight discomfort without causing pain. Encourage patients to communicate their sensations, as this feedback will help tailor the pressure and duration of future sessions.

Tips for beginners to avoid common mistakes

Beginners in auriculotherapy should prioritize education and practice to minimize mistakes. Familiarize yourself with ear anatomy and the location of key acupuncture points before beginning treatments. Use diagrams and models for reference, and consider attending workshops or classes to enhance your skills. Practice inserting needles on practice mats or with supervision until you feel confident.

Additionally, ensure you're using the right tools and maintaining hygiene. Double-check that your needles and equipment are sterile and that your treatment space is clean. Encourage patients to share their feelings and experiences during treatment to better understand their responses. Learning from each session will significantly improve your techniques and patient outcomes over time.

How to observe patient responses during the session

During the auriculotherapy session, it's essential to closely observe the patient's physical and emotional responses. Look for non-verbal cues such as facial expressions, body language, and any signs of discomfort or relaxation. Encourage patients to vocalize their feelings about the treatment, which can provide valuable insights into their experience and help you adjust accordingly.

You can also ask specific questions about their sensations during treatment, such as whether they feel any tingling or warmth in the treated areas. Document these observations and any patient feedback, as this information will be crucial for tailoring future treatments and enhancing overall efficacy.

Proper aftercare for treated ear points

After completing an auriculotherapy session, it's important to provide proper aftercare instructions to the patient. Advise them to avoid touching or manipulating the treated areas to prevent irritation or infection. If needles were used, instruct the patient to keep the area clean and dry, and remind them not to engage in any strenuous activities that could disturb the treated points for at least 24 hours.

For those using ear seeds, remind them to avoid excessive moisture and to change the seeds if they become loose or fall off. Suggest light pressure on the seeds for added stimulation and provide guidance on how often to reapply or change them. Follow-up with the patient to address any concerns and reinforce the importance of maintaining the benefits of the treatment.

Understanding patient feedback and adjusting treatments

Listening to patient feedback is vital for effective auriculotherapy. After each session, ask open-ended questions to gain insights into their experiences and any changes they've noticed in their symptoms. This dialogue helps establish trust and encourages patients to share their feelings, making it easier to adjust treatments based on their responses.

Based on the feedback received, be prepared to modify your approach for future sessions. This may involve changing needle placement, adjusting pressure levels, or altering the frequency of treatments. Continuous communication ensures that the therapy remains aligned with the patient's needs and enhances the overall effectiveness of the treatment plan.

Methods for combining auriculotherapy with body acupuncture

Combining auriculotherapy with body acupuncture can enhance treatment outcomes. Begin by assessing the patient's overall condition and identifying specific areas of concern that may benefit from both methods. Use ear acupuncture for targeted relief of symptoms while simultaneously addressing underlying issues through body points.

When planning a combined session, introduce the ear acupuncture first to establish a baseline response. Follow this with body acupuncture, taking care to monitor the patient's reactions throughout. By integrating both approaches, you can provide a holistic treatment that addresses physical, emotional, and energetic imbalances in a comprehensive manner.

Recommended frequency of sessions for different conditions

The frequency of auriculotherapy sessions depends on the specific condition being treated. For acute issues such as pain relief, patients may benefit from 2 to 3 sessions per week until symptoms improve. Chronic conditions might require weekly sessions, with the possibility of gradually reducing frequency as the patient progresses.

Always personalize the treatment schedule based on the patient's response and feedback. Regularly assess the effectiveness of the therapy and be open to adjusting the frequency as necessary. By maintaining flexibility in your approach, you can better accommodate the patient's evolving needs and enhance their overall treatment experience.

Dos and don'ts of treating sensitive or inflamed ears

When treating sensitive or inflamed ears, it's crucial to approach the situation with care. Do consult with the patient about any history of ear problems and conduct a thorough examination of the affected area. Always use clean, sterile needles and minimize pressure on sensitive points to avoid causing further discomfort.

Don't attempt to treat areas that show signs of severe infection or trauma without consulting a healthcare professional. Avoid using acupuncture needles in inflamed areas until they have healed. Instead, consider using acupressure techniques or ear seeds for a gentler approach. By respecting the patient's sensitivity, you can ensure a safer and more effective treatment experience.

How to track treatment progress over multiple sessions

Tracking treatment progress is essential to evaluate the effectiveness of auriculotherapy. Begin by documenting each session, including details such as the specific points treated, techniques used, and patient feedback. This log will help you identify patterns, improvements, or setbacks over time, enabling you to adjust treatments accordingly.

Encourage patients to maintain a journal of their symptoms and any changes they experience between sessions. This self-monitoring can provide valuable insights into the long-term effects of treatment and foster a deeper understanding of their progress. Regularly review this information together to create a collaborative approach to their healing journey.

CHAPTER 5:

Treating Common Ailments with Auriculotherapy

Pain Relief Techniques for Back and Neck Pain

To alleviate back and neck pain through auriculotherapy, first identify the specific ear points associated with these areas, such as the cervical spine point and the lumbar spine point. Using a specialized ear acupuncture needle or small seeds, gently stimulate these points for a few seconds. This technique can help release tension, improve blood circulation, and promote the body's natural healing process.

Additionally, combining this method with heat therapy can enhance pain relief. Apply a warm compress to the affected areas after stimulating the ear points, allowing for deeper relaxation. Regularly practicing this technique, ideally under the guidance of a trained practitioner, can lead to significant improvements in pain management.

Treating Headaches and Migraines through Ear Points

Ear acupuncture offers effective relief for headaches and migraines by targeting specific auricular points, such as the head point and the occipital point. To practice this technique, locate these points on the ear and gently apply pressure or insert needles. This stimulation encourages the release of endorphins, which act as natural painkillers, reducing headache intensity.

For optimal results, consider pairing this method with lifestyle changes like hydration and stress management. Keeping a headache diary to identify triggers can also help refine your approach. Over time, regular treatment can significantly decrease the frequency and severity of headaches.

Reducing Stress and Anxiety with Ear Acupuncture

Auriculotherapy is a powerful tool for managing stress and anxiety. Start by locating the calming points on the ear, such as the shen men point and the autonomic nervous system point. Stimulating these areas can help promote relaxation and balance within the body's systems, making it easier to cope with everyday stressors.

To enhance the effects, incorporate deep breathing exercises during your sessions. Focusing on your breath while applying pressure to the ear points can deepen relaxation. Regular sessions, whether self-administered or with a professional, can lead to a more profound sense of calm and emotional stability.

Managing Digestive Issues Such as Indigestion and IBS

For digestive issues like indigestion and IBS, auriculotherapy can be a helpful complementary treatment. Key points to focus on include the stomach and small intestine points located on the ear. By gently stimulating these areas, you can encourage improved digestive function and alleviate discomfort.

Incorporating lifestyle modifications, such as mindful eating and stress reduction, alongside ear acupuncture can enhance results. Keeping a food diary to track symptoms can also be beneficial, allowing you to identify specific triggers and adjust your diet accordingly.

Ear Points for Alleviating Menstrual Cramps and Hormone Imbalances

Auriculotherapy can effectively reduce menstrual cramps and address hormone imbalances. Identify the relevant ear points, such as the uterus and endocrine points, and stimulate them using gentle pressure or needles. This stimulation can help relieve pain and regulate hormonal fluctuations, leading to a more comfortable menstrual cycle.

Additionally, consider combining ear acupuncture with herbal remedies or dietary changes to support hormonal balance. Engaging in regular exercise can also alleviate symptoms and promote overall well-being during your menstrual cycle.

Techniques for Improving Sleep and Treating Insomnia

To improve sleep and combat insomnia through auriculotherapy, focus on the sleep point and the shen men point on the ear. Gently stimulate these points for several minutes before bedtime to promote relaxation and prepare your body for sleep. This technique can help reduce the time it takes to fall asleep and enhance sleep quality.

Creating a calming bedtime routine that includes ear acupuncture can further support better sleep. Incorporate activities like reading or meditation to wind down before sleep, allowing the effects of the ear stimulation to work in tandem with your efforts to achieve restful slumber.

Reducing Symptoms of Allergies and Sinusitis

Auriculotherapy can also aid in managing allergy symptoms and sinusitis. Target key points such as the sinus and allergy points on the ear, applying gentle pressure or acupuncture needles. This stimulation can help reduce inflammation and enhance the body's immune response, providing relief from common allergy symptoms.

For added benefit, consider using essential oils or herbal remedies known for their anti-inflammatory properties alongside your ear acupuncture sessions. Regular practice can help decrease the severity and frequency of allergic reactions over time.

Ear Acupuncture for Boosting Energy and Vitality

To boost energy and vitality, focus on stimulating the energy points located on the ear, such as the adrenal gland point. By applying pressure or using acupuncture techniques on these areas, you can stimulate the body's natural energy production, reducing feelings of fatigue and lethargy.

Incorporating regular physical activity and a balanced diet can complement the effects of ear acupuncture. This combination promotes overall health and well-being, ensuring that your body has the energy it needs to function optimally.

Treating Addiction and Managing Withdrawal Symptoms

Auriculotherapy can be a valuable aid in treating addiction and managing withdrawal symptoms. Identify the addiction and withdrawal points on the ear, such as the addiction point and the calming point. By stimulating these areas, you can help reduce cravings and anxiety, making it easier to cope with withdrawal.

Combining ear acupuncture with counseling and support groups enhances its effectiveness. This comprehensive approach can provide a well-rounded strategy for recovery, promoting both physical and emotional healing.

Auriculotherapy for Chronic Fatigue and Fibromyalgia

For those suffering from chronic fatigue and fibromyalgia, auriculotherapy offers a potential avenue for relief. Focus on stimulating points related to fatigue and pain management on the ear. Regular stimulation can help reduce pain and improve overall energy levels, contributing to a better quality of life.

Incorporating relaxation techniques such as yoga or meditation can complement ear acupuncture. This holistic approach can lead to significant improvements in both physical and mental well-being for individuals dealing with chronic conditions.

Techniques for Managing Arthritis and Joint Pain

Managing arthritis and joint pain through auriculotherapy involves targeting specific ear points, such as the joint and pain points. Gently stimulate these areas to promote pain relief and reduce inflammation in affected joints. Regular sessions can help enhance mobility and decrease discomfort over time.

In conjunction with ear acupuncture, maintaining a healthy weight and engaging in low-impact exercise can provide further relief. This multi-faceted approach ensures that you address both the symptoms and underlying causes of arthritis effectively.

Ear Points for Improving Focus and Mental Clarity

To improve focus and mental clarity, auriculotherapy can be beneficial. Locate and stimulate ear points associated with mental function, such as the brain point and the cerebellum point. This practice can enhance cognitive function, helping to sharpen focus and improve overall mental performance.

Additionally, incorporating mindfulness techniques and regular breaks during study or work sessions can maximize the benefits of ear acupuncture. This combination fosters a conducive environment for improved concentration and productivity.

Addressing Emotional Trauma and Mental Health Disorders

Auriculotherapy can play a significant role in addressing emotional trauma and mental health disorders. By targeting points associated with emotional well-being, such as the emotional balance point and the shen men point, you can promote healing and stability. Regularly practicing this technique can help alleviate symptoms of anxiety, depression, and PTSD.

Combining ear acupuncture with therapy or support groups can enhance the healing process. This integrated approach ensures that you address both the emotional and psychological aspects of trauma, fostering a more holistic path to recovery.

Identifying Patients Who Should Avoid Ear Acupuncture

Before administering ear acupuncture, it's crucial to identify patients who should avoid this treatment. Individuals with bleeding disorders, such as hemophilia, should not undergo ear acupuncture due to the risk of excessive bleeding. Additionally, those who have recently undergone surgery or have active infections in the ear area should be evaluated carefully before proceeding.

Other individuals to consider include those with severe allergies to metals or silicone, which could be present in the acupuncture needles or ear beads. Pregnant women and those with certain chronic health conditions, like autoimmune disorders, should also be assessed for potential risks before treatment.

Recognizing Signs of Allergic Reactions to Materials Used

Allergic reactions to materials used in ear acupuncture can manifest in various ways. Patients may experience redness, itching, swelling, or a rash at the site of needle insertion. It's essential for practitioners to be vigilant and inquire about any known allergies before beginning treatment.

If a patient exhibits signs of an allergic reaction during or after a session, the practitioner should immediately remove the needles and apply a cold compress to alleviate symptoms. In more severe cases, it may be necessary to seek medical attention if symptoms persist or escalate.

Safety Guidelines for Pregnant Women and Children

Ear acupuncture can be beneficial for pregnant women, but specific safety guidelines should be followed. It's advisable to avoid certain ear points that may stimulate uterine contractions. Always consult with a healthcare provider before starting treatment to ensure it is safe for both the mother and fetus.

For children, special considerations should be made regarding needle size and technique. Practitioners should use smaller needles and maintain a gentle approach to minimize discomfort. It's also essential to explain the procedure to both the child and their guardians to ease anxiety and build trust.

Contraindications for Individuals with Pacemakers

Patients with pacemakers should avoid ear acupuncture, particularly at specific ear points that could interfere with the device's functioning. It's important to assess the patient's medical history thoroughly and consult with their cardiologist if there's any uncertainty regarding treatment.

When working with patients who have pacemakers, practitioners must ensure that needles are placed away from the vagus nerve area, which could potentially disrupt heart rhythms. Educating patients on the risks involved can help them make informed decisions about their treatment options.

How to Handle Infections or Skin Irritation at Ear Points

If a patient presents with infections or skin irritations at ear points, ear acupuncture should be postponed until the issue is resolved. Practitioners should assess the area for signs of inflammation, pus, or severe redness before proceeding with treatment.

In case of irritation, gentle cleaning with antiseptic solutions may help reduce symptoms. If the irritation or infection persists, practitioners should recommend that patients consult a healthcare professional for further evaluation and treatment.

Proper Needle Disposal and Infection Prevention

Proper needle disposal is critical for preventing infections in ear acupuncture practices. Practitioners should use designated sharps containers for used needles to ensure safe disposal. Avoid recapping needles after use, as this increases the risk of injury.

Infection prevention also involves maintaining a clean environment. Practitioners should wash their hands thoroughly before and after each session and use sterile needles. Cleaning and disinfecting surfaces and equipment regularly can further minimize the risk of infection.

Ear Conditions That May Complicate Treatment

Certain ear conditions can complicate ear acupuncture treatment. Patients with conditions such as severe ear infections, perforated eardrums, or chronic otitis media should be assessed carefully. If a patient has active ear conditions, it may be best to delay acupuncture until they have been resolved.

Practitioners should also monitor for complications such as swelling or pain during treatment. If these occur, it's important to stop the session and evaluate whether to proceed or refer the patient to a specialist for further care.

Recognizing When to Refer Patients to a Medical Professional

Practitioners should be skilled in recognizing when a patient requires referral to a medical professional. Signs that warrant referral include persistent pain, unusual swelling, or complications from underlying medical conditions. If a patient's condition does not improve after a few sessions, it may indicate the need for further medical evaluation.

Furthermore, if a patient presents with symptoms that are beyond the scope of ear acupuncture, such as significant hearing loss or dizziness, it's crucial to guide them to an appropriate healthcare provider. This not only ensures patient safety but also helps maintain a professional standard of care.

Legal Regulations and Licensing Requirements for Practitioners

Practitioners of ear acupuncture must be aware of legal regulations and licensing requirements that vary by region. Obtaining the necessary certifications and licenses is essential to practice legally and ethically. Research local laws to ensure compliance with regulations related to acupuncture practices.

Practitioners should also be familiar with the scope of practice in their area to avoid legal issues. Participating in ongoing education and training helps practitioners stay informed about any changes in regulations and enhances their skills.

Best Practices for Ensuring Patient Safety During Sessions

Ensuring patient safety during ear acupuncture sessions is paramount. Practitioners should maintain a calm and clean environment, utilizing sterile equipment and providing clear instructions to patients. Before starting, it's essential to perform a thorough assessment and confirm the patient's medical history.

During the session, practitioners should monitor the patient closely for any signs of discomfort or distress. Establishing open communication with patients encourages them to express concerns, allowing practitioners to address any issues promptly and adjust treatment as needed.

Guidelines for Handling Patient Discomfort or Pain

Handling patient discomfort during ear acupuncture requires sensitivity and immediate attention. Practitioners should ask for feedback throughout the session and be attentive to verbal and non-verbal cues. If a patient reports pain, the practitioner should assess the needle placement and make adjustments accordingly.

In cases of significant discomfort, practitioners should stop the treatment and discuss alternative methods or adjust the technique. Educating patients on what to expect can also help alleviate anxiety and minimize discomfort during the session.

Managing Needle Phobia and Patient Anxiety

Managing needle phobia and patient anxiety is essential for a positive ear acupuncture experience. Practitioners should take the time to explain the procedure and benefits thoroughly, allowing patients to ask questions. Demonstrating the equipment and providing reassurance can help build trust.

Using relaxation techniques such as deep breathing or visualization can also assist in calming anxious patients. Practitioners might consider offering treatment in a comfortable, quiet space, as this can further reduce anxiety and create a more positive environment.

Addressing Issues of Dizziness or Fainting During Treatments

Dizziness or fainting during ear acupuncture treatments can occur, especially in sensitive individuals. If a patient experiences these symptoms, it's essential to have them lie down in a safe position, preferably with their legs elevated. Practitioners should monitor their condition closely and offer water or a light snack to help stabilize them.

Preventative measures include assessing patients for any prior history of dizziness or fainting. Encouraging patients to avoid heavy meals or strenuous activity before their session can also reduce the likelihood of these occurrences, creating a safer experience overall

CHAPTER 7:

Combining Auriculotherapy with Other Therapies

Integrating Auriculotherapy with Body Acupuncture

Integrating auriculotherapy with body acupuncture can enhance the overall therapeutic experience. By targeting specific points on the ear, practitioners can address systemic issues while also working on local body acupuncture points. For instance, if a patient is experiencing lower back pain, applying ear acupuncture on points related to the back can amplify the treatment's effectiveness and promote faster healing.

To effectively combine these modalities, practitioners should first assess the patient's condition and then determine which auricular points to stimulate alongside the body acupuncture points. Utilizing both techniques during a single session can lead to a more comprehensive treatment plan, ensuring that both the localized and systemic aspects of the patient's health are addressed.

Combining Ear Acupuncture with Herbal Remedies

Combining ear acupuncture with herbal remedies can significantly enhance treatment outcomes. Herbal remedies can be used to support the effects of auriculotherapy by providing the body with essential nutrients and compounds that promote healing. Practitioners can recommend specific herbal formulas based on the patient's unique needs and the conditions being treated, ensuring a holistic approach.

To implement this combination, practitioners should evaluate the patient's specific health issues and then suggest appropriate herbal remedies that complement the ear acupuncture treatment. This can involve administering herbal teas, tinctures, or capsules that align with the goals of the acupuncture session, creating a synergistic effect that promotes healing and well-being.

How Auriculotherapy Complements Massage Therapy

Auriculotherapy can serve as a powerful adjunct to massage therapy by addressing underlying issues that may be contributing to muscle tension and pain. By stimulating specific points on the ear, practitioners can help relieve stress, enhance relaxation, and promote a deeper healing experience during the massage. This approach can lead to improved patient outcomes, as the body can release tension more effectively.

For optimal results, massage therapists can coordinate with acupuncturists to integrate auriculotherapy into the treatment plan. This can be achieved by applying ear acupuncture before or during a massage session to address pain points or tension areas, thereby enhancing the overall therapeutic effects and providing the patient with a more comprehensive care experience.

Using Ear Acupuncture Alongside Chiropractic Care

Ear acupuncture can complement chiropractic care by addressing issues such as pain management, stress reduction, and muscle relaxation. By targeting specific auricular points, practitioners can help patients experience enhanced relief from discomfort, making chiropractic adjustments more effective. This combination can provide a holistic approach to spinal health and overall wellness.

To successfully incorporate ear acupuncture into chiropractic care, chiropractors can assess the patient's spinal issues and recommend auriculotherapy to be performed either before or after spinal adjustments. This approach can enhance the patient's overall experience by addressing both the physical alignment of the spine and the underlying tension that may contribute to discomfort.

Techniques for Combining Ear Acupuncture with Moxibustion

Moxibustion, the practice of burning mugwort on or near acupuncture points, can be effectively combined with ear acupuncture to enhance therapeutic outcomes. This technique warms and invigorates the qi (energy) at targeted points, promoting better circulation and relieving pain. Practitioners can use moxibustion on ear points that correspond to areas of discomfort in the body, maximizing the benefits of both modalities.

To apply this technique, practitioners should first perform ear acupuncture to establish the desired effects. Afterward, moxibustion can be applied to the corresponding auricular points. This combination creates a warming effect that can help to deepen relaxation and increase the efficacy of the treatment, allowing patients to experience greater relief from their symptoms.

Pairing Ear Acupuncture with Mindfulness and Meditation Practices

Integrating mindfulness and meditation with ear acupuncture can enhance the mental and emotional benefits of the treatment. Ear acupuncture can help calm the nervous system and promote relaxation, setting the stage for a more profound mindfulness practice. By incorporating mindfulness techniques during the acupuncture session, patients can experience heightened awareness and emotional clarity.

Practitioners can guide patients in mindfulness exercises during their auriculotherapy sessions. Techniques such as focused breathing, body scans, or visualization can be introduced alongside ear acupuncture. This approach helps patients deepen their relaxation experience, allowing them to connect with their bodies and emotions in a meaningful way, leading to overall wellness.

How to Incorporate Essential Oils in Auriculotherapy Sessions

Incorporating essential oils into auriculotherapy can enhance the treatment experience and promote healing through aromatherapy. Essential oils possess various therapeutic properties, such as pain relief and stress reduction, which can complement the effects of ear acupuncture. Practitioners can use oils like lavender for relaxation or peppermint for invigorating energy, depending on the patient's needs.

To use essential oils, practitioners should apply a few drops of diluted oil to the auricular points before or after the acupuncture session. This can be done by gently massaging the oil onto the ear or using a diffuser in the treatment space. The combination of essential oils with auriculotherapy not only enhances the healing effects but also creates a soothing atmosphere for the patient.

Combining Ear Acupuncture with Diet and Lifestyle Changes

Integrating dietary and lifestyle changes with ear acupuncture can lead to more effective and sustainable health improvements. Practitioners can provide patients with personalized recommendations based on their specific health conditions, addressing underlying issues that may contribute to their ailments. This holistic approach emphasizes the importance of nutrition and lifestyle in achieving optimal health.

To implement this combination, practitioners should discuss the patient's dietary habits and lifestyle choices during the initial consultation. After assessing the patient's needs, they can recommend specific changes that align with their ear acupuncture treatment, such as increasing hydration, incorporating more whole foods, or establishing a regular exercise routine. This multi-faceted approach ensures patients receive comprehensive support on their healing journey.

Using Ear Seeds to Prolong Effects After Acupuncture Sessions

Ear seeds are small seeds or beads placed on specific auricular points to prolong the effects of ear acupuncture. They serve as a form of self-acupuncture that patients can use at home, helping to maintain the benefits of their treatment between sessions. This technique can enhance the healing process and empower patients to take an active role in their wellness.

To use ear seeds, practitioners should apply them to targeted auricular points at the end of an acupuncture session. Patients can then be instructed on how to press the seeds gently throughout the day, stimulating the points and reinforcing the treatment's effects. This practice not only aids in pain relief but also encourages mindfulness and awareness of the body.

Collaborating with Other Healthcare Professionals

Collaboration among healthcare professionals can enhance patient outcomes in auriculotherapy. Practitioners can work alongside medical doctors, physical therapists, and nutritionists to create comprehensive treatment plans tailored to individual patient needs. This integrated approach allows for a more holistic view of patient care, addressing multiple aspects of health and well-being.

To facilitate collaboration, practitioners should communicate openly with other healthcare professionals involved in a patient's care. This may include sharing treatment goals, progress updates, and any relevant findings from auriculotherapy sessions. By fostering teamwork among various practitioners, patients can receive cohesive and effective treatment, leading to improved health results.

Treating Chronic Conditions with a Multi-Therapy Approach

A multi-therapy approach using auriculotherapy can be particularly effective in managing chronic conditions. By combining ear acupuncture with other modalities such as physical therapy, medication, or counseling, practitioners can address the complex nature of chronic illnesses and enhance the patient's quality of life. This integrated method allows for comprehensive care tailored to the patient's unique circumstances.

To implement this approach, practitioners should first assess the patient's chronic condition and identify potential complementary therapies. This might involve coordinating with other healthcare providers to ensure a cohesive treatment plan. By incorporating multiple therapies, patients can experience improved symptom management and a greater sense of empowerment in their healing journey.

The Role of Ear Acupuncture in Postoperative Care

Ear acupuncture can play a significant role in postoperative care by promoting healing, reducing pain, and alleviating anxiety. This approach can help patients recover more comfortably and speed up their healing process. By addressing both physical and emotional needs, auriculotherapy can enhance the overall experience of recovery.

To utilize ear acupuncture in postoperative care, practitioners should assess the patient's surgical history and pain levels. They can then stimulate specific auricular points that correspond to pain management and relaxation, providing immediate relief and supporting the body's natural healing processes. This proactive approach can lead to better patient satisfaction and improved surgical outcomes.

Ear Acupuncture for Enhancing Overall Wellness

Ear acupuncture can be a valuable tool for enhancing overall wellness and promoting a balanced lifestyle. By addressing physical, emotional, and mental health issues, auriculotherapy can help individuals achieve a greater sense of well-being. Regular ear acupuncture sessions can support stress management, improve sleep quality, and boost energy levels.

To promote wellness through ear acupuncture, practitioners can encourage patients to incorporate regular sessions into their self-care routines. By assessing individual health goals and needs, practitioners can create tailored treatment plans that address specific concerns. This holistic approach empowers patients to take charge of their health and fosters long-term wellness.

CHAPTER 8:

Common Concerns and FAQs in Auriculotherapy

Does Auriculotherapy Hurt, and How Long Do Sessions Last?

Auriculotherapy typically causes minimal discomfort. Most individuals report a mild sensation during the insertion of the needles, often described as a slight tingling or pressure. The discomfort is generally short-lived, and many find the experience relaxing. Sessions usually last between 20 to 40 minutes, allowing adequate time for stimulation of the ear points.

To ensure comfort, it's important to communicate with your practitioner about any pain thresholds or anxieties you may have. If you're nervous, consider starting with shorter sessions to build your comfort level. This can help you ease into the process while receiving effective treatment.

How Many Treatments Are Necessary to See Results?

The number of treatments required can vary depending on the individual's condition and response to therapy. Generally, clients may start to see results after 3 to 5 sessions, but some conditions may require 8 to 12 treatments to achieve optimal effects. Your practitioner will tailor a treatment plan based on your specific needs and progress.

Consistency is key in auriculotherapy. Attending sessions regularly will enhance the benefits, as the cumulative effects of treatment often lead to more significant pain relief and improved well-being over time.

What Are the Risks or Side Effects of Ear Acupuncture?

Auriculotherapy is generally safe when performed by a qualified practitioner, but some mild side effects can occur. These may include slight bruising, soreness at the needle insertion points, or temporary dizziness. Most side effects are minor and resolve quickly.

It's crucial to choose a licensed acupuncturist who follows strict hygiene practices. This minimizes risks such as infections or adverse reactions. Always discuss any concerns or medical conditions with your practitioner before starting treatment.

Can Auriculotherapy Be Self-Administered at Home?

Yes, auriculotherapy can be self-administered with proper guidance. Many practitioners provide training on how to locate ear points and use self-adhesive seeds or beads that can stimulate specific areas. It's essential to follow instructions closely to ensure effectiveness and avoid injury.

Begin by familiarizing yourself with the ear anatomy and the specific points that correspond to your needs. Start with short sessions, paying attention to how your body responds, and adjust as necessary for comfort and effectiveness.

How Does Ear Acupuncture Compare to Body Acupuncture?

Ear acupuncture targets specific points on the ear that correspond to different areas of the body, making it a focused approach. While both methods aim to balance energy and relieve pain, ear acupuncture often addresses issues more quickly due to the ear's extensive nerve connections.

Practitioners may recommend combining both techniques for a comprehensive treatment plan. Using body acupuncture alongside auriculotherapy can enhance overall results, addressing both local and systemic issues simultaneously.

Is Ear Acupuncture Effective for Weight Loss or Addiction?

Research suggests that auriculotherapy can be effective for weight loss and addiction. It works by stimulating points associated with appetite control, cravings, and stress relief. Regular sessions can help support individuals in their journey to modify behaviors and achieve their goals.

To optimize results, consider combining auriculotherapy with lifestyle changes like diet and exercise or behavioral therapy. A holistic approach tends to yield the best outcomes, ensuring long-term success in weight management or overcoming addiction.

Can Ear Acupuncture Treat Emotional or Psychological Issues?

Yes, auriculotherapy has been shown to address emotional and psychological issues, such as anxiety and depression. By stimulating specific points on the ear, it can promote relaxation and emotional balance. Many practitioners report that clients experience reduced stress and improved mood following treatments.

For those seeking to manage emotional health, regular sessions can enhance mental clarity and emotional resilience. It is advisable to work with a qualified practitioner to develop a tailored approach that includes supportive therapies.

What Should I Do If a Point Feels Sore or Tender After Treatment?

If you experience soreness or tenderness at a treatment point, it's essential to take care of the area. Applying a cold compress can reduce swelling and discomfort. Additionally, you may want to avoid touching or irritating the area for a short period.

Communicate with your practitioner about any soreness you experience. They can provide advice on managing discomfort and may adjust future treatments based on your feedback, ensuring a more comfortable experience going forward.

How Can I Ensure Accuracy When Locating Ear Points?

Accuracy in locating ear points is crucial for effective auriculotherapy. Use a reliable ear acupuncture chart to identify points relevant to your condition. Practice regularly and consider seeking guidance from a certified practitioner for hands-on training.

In addition, you can use tools such as ear models or diagrams to familiarize yourself with anatomical landmarks. Taking your time to learn and practice will enhance your confidence in identifying the correct points for self-treatment.

Can Ear Acupuncture Be Combined with Medication or Other Therapies?

Auriculotherapy can be safely combined with medications and other therapeutic modalities. It is often used as a complementary treatment, enhancing the effects of prescribed medications or therapies without interference. Always inform your healthcare provider about all treatments you are receiving.

This integrative approach can lead to more comprehensive health management. For instance, combining ear acupuncture with physical therapy can provide relief from pain while promoting healing, making it a valuable addition to your care regimen.

What Is the Best Frequency for Auriculotherapy Treatments?

The optimal frequency for auriculotherapy treatments typically depends on the condition being treated. For chronic issues, weekly sessions may be recommended initially, gradually decreasing to bi-weekly or monthly sessions as improvements are noticed.

Your practitioner will assess your progress and adjust the frequency accordingly. Maintaining open communication about your experiences will help determine the best treatment schedule for your needs.

How Should I Care for My Ears After a Session?

Post-treatment ear care is simple but essential. Avoid exposing your ears to harsh environments, such as extreme heat or cold, and refrain from inserting objects into the ear canal for a few days. Keeping the area clean will help prevent irritation or infection.

Additionally, if you have received ear beads or seeds, follow your practitioner's instructions on their care and maintenance. Regular checks will ensure they remain in place and effective in stimulating the points until your next session.

Is Auriculotherapy Safe for Children and the Elderly?

Auriculotherapy is generally safe for both children and the elderly, though modifications may be necessary based on individual health conditions. Pediatric patients often respond well to this therapy, and practitioners can adjust the techniques to suit younger clients.

For elderly patients, it's essential to consider any underlying health issues and adjust treatment plans accordingly. Consulting with a qualified practitioner will help ensure safe and effective treatment for all age groups.

CHAPTER 9:

Advanced Techniques and Future Developments

Overview of Advanced Needle Techniques for Experienced Practitioners

Experienced practitioners in auriculotherapy can enhance their skills through advanced needle techniques, which include different insertion angles, depths, and techniques such as "Sham Needle" techniques that allow for the practice of needle placement without puncturing the skin. Learning how to manipulate needles to stimulate specific points effectively can maximize therapeutic outcomes. Practitioners may also explore techniques like intradermal needling, where small needles are placed just under the skin for prolonged stimulation.

In practice, advanced techniques require a thorough understanding of ear anatomy and the specific points relevant to various conditions. Practitioners should utilize these advanced techniques while maintaining patient comfort and safety. Proper hygiene and technique will minimize discomfort and enhance the healing process, enabling practitioners to tailor treatments to individual patient needs and conditions.

Using Electrical Stimulation for Deeper Results

Electrical stimulation can significantly enhance the effects of ear acupuncture by providing continuous stimulation to acupoints, which may lead to deeper and longer-lasting results. Practitioners can use devices that deliver low-frequency electrical impulses to the needles already placed in the ear. This method increases blood circulation and promotes tissue repair while reducing pain perception.

To implement this technique, practitioners should begin with standard needle insertion into the acupoints before attaching the electrical stimulation device. It's essential to start with lower frequencies to assess patient tolerance before gradually increasing intensity. Practitioners must ensure that the device is well-maintained and the settings adjusted based on individual patient feedback for optimal results.

Incorporating Laser Therapy into Auriculotherapy Practices

Laser therapy can be an effective, non-invasive addition to auriculotherapy, employing low-level lasers (cold lasers) to stimulate acupoints without the need for needles. This method is especially beneficial for patients who are needle-phobic or have conditions where traditional needling may not be suitable. Practitioners can use handheld laser devices to target specific ear points, promoting healing through photobiomodulation.

To incorporate laser therapy, practitioners should familiarize themselves with the specific parameters of their laser device, including power output and treatment duration. Targeting specific auricular points with the laser for about 30 seconds to a minute per point can yield beneficial results. Practitioners should also educate patients on the benefits and safety of this method to encourage its acceptance.

Emerging Research in Auriculotherapy for Chronic Diseases

Recent studies have explored the potential of auriculotherapy in managing chronic diseases such as diabetes, hypertension, and chronic pain conditions. Emerging research suggests that stimulating specific ear points may help regulate hormonal responses, reduce inflammation, and promote overall health. Practitioners should stay abreast of these findings to provide evidence-based treatments that resonate with patient needs.

For practical application, practitioners should consider integrating auriculotherapy as a complementary approach within a broader treatment plan for chronic conditions. Documenting patient outcomes related to auriculotherapy can help practitioners refine their techniques and adapt treatments based on individual responses. Collaboration with other healthcare professionals can enhance the holistic approach to chronic disease management.

How to Expand Your Practice with New Ear Acupuncture Tools

Investing in new tools and technologies can elevate an auriculotherapy practice, enabling practitioners to offer a broader range of services. Essential tools may include advanced needle types, electrical stimulation devices, or laser equipment. These innovations not only improve treatment efficacy but can also attract new clients interested in cutting-edge therapies.

To implement these tools effectively, practitioners should undergo training specific to each device's usage and safety protocols. Regular workshops and hands-on practice can build confidence in using new techniques. Promoting these expanded services through marketing strategies can increase visibility and draw in clients seeking modern approaches to ear acupuncture.

Developments in Auriculotherapy Technology and Devices

Technological advancements have greatly enhanced the field of auriculotherapy, with the development of devices that allow for precision stimulation and better patient comfort. Innovations such as programmable electrical stimulation machines or wireless laser devices facilitate treatment customization for various patient needs. Practitioners should explore these technologies to stay competitive and offer the best care possible.

When integrating new devices into practice, practitioners must prioritize proper training to understand the operational intricacies and safety measures associated with each tool. Creating protocols for their application can streamline the integration process and ensure consistent results. Ongoing assessment of the effectiveness of these devices will further refine treatment strategies and patient outcomes.

Ear Acupuncture for Treating Emotional Trauma and PTSD

Ear acupuncture has emerged as a valuable therapeutic tool for individuals dealing with emotional trauma and PTSD. Targeting specific points on the ear can help regulate the nervous system, alleviate anxiety, and promote emotional healing. Practitioners should approach treatment with sensitivity, creating a supportive environment that encourages patient openness.

To apply ear acupuncture for these issues, practitioners typically focus on points associated with calming the mind and body, such as the Shen Men and sympathetic nervous system points. Initial sessions may involve gentle stimulation with needles or laser therapy, followed by discussions on emotional experiences. Establishing a trusting rapport with patients will enhance the treatment's effectiveness and encourage ongoing participation in their healing journey.

Auriculotherapy in Palliative and Cancer Care

Auriculotherapy can play a significant role in palliative care, providing pain relief and improving quality of life for cancer patients. By targeting specific auricular points, practitioners can help manage symptoms such as pain, nausea, and anxiety often associated with cancer treatments. The approach can be tailored to each patient's unique symptoms, offering a holistic adjunct to conventional care.

In practice, practitioners should conduct thorough assessments to identify the most relevant acupoints for each patient. Combining auriculotherapy with other supportive therapies can enhance its effectiveness. Regular follow-ups and adjustments to treatment protocols based on patient feedback are essential for optimizing care in palliative settings.

The Future Role of Ear Acupuncture in Holistic Medicine

The future of auriculotherapy looks promising as it gains recognition within holistic medicine frameworks. As more healthcare providers acknowledge the importance of integrative therapies, ear acupuncture is increasingly being included in treatment protocols. This trend underscores the growing acceptance of non-invasive modalities in managing various health conditions.

To prepare for this shift, practitioners should continue to enhance their knowledge and skills in auriculotherapy. Engaging in interdisciplinary collaborations with other health professionals can provide valuable insights and broaden treatment options for patients. Practitioners should also consider participating in research studies to contribute to the body of evidence supporting auriculotherapy's efficacy in holistic health.

New Studies and Findings on the Effectiveness of Auriculotherapy

Recent research has provided new insights into the effectiveness of auriculotherapy for various conditions, reinforcing its potential as a therapeutic intervention. Studies indicate significant positive outcomes in pain management, addiction treatment, and stress reduction. Staying informed about these developments allows practitioners to incorporate current evidence into their practice.

Practitioners can actively seek out and review new studies published in journals dedicated to complementary and alternative medicine. Integrating findings from these studies into patient care can enhance treatment strategies and provide patients with a sense of confidence in their treatment plan. Regularly discussing relevant research during patient consultations can also help educate patients about the benefits of auriculotherapy.

How to Stay Updated on Advancements in the Field

Staying updated on advancements in auriculotherapy is crucial for practitioners seeking to enhance their skills and treatment offerings. Regularly attending workshops, webinars, and conferences focused on auriculotherapy can provide valuable insights into emerging techniques and research findings. Networking with other practitioners can also foster knowledge sharing and professional growth.

To maintain current knowledge, practitioners should subscribe to relevant journals, join professional organizations, and participate in online forums dedicated to auriculotherapy. Continuous education and active engagement in the professional community will help practitioners stay at the forefront of advancements in the field and ultimately improve patient care.

Certification Programs for Advanced Auriculotherapy Training

Enrolling in certification programs for advanced auriculotherapy training can significantly enhance a practitioner's credentials and expertise. These programs typically offer comprehensive education on advanced techniques, including needle techniques, electrical stimulation, and laser therapy. Completing such programs can elevate a practitioner's practice and increase their marketability.

To find suitable certification programs, practitioners should research accredited organizations that offer specialized training in auriculotherapy. Prioritizing hands-on training opportunities within these programs can enhance practical skills. Additionally, networking with fellow practitioners during these programs can provide valuable insights and foster professional relationships that benefit future practice.

Ways to Expand Your Practice through Continuing Education

Continuing education is vital for practitioners looking to expand their auriculotherapy practice. Pursuing additional certifications, attending workshops, and engaging in relevant online courses can introduce new techniques and perspectives that enhance patient care. This commitment to learning can also distinguish practitioners in a competitive market.

Practitioners should identify areas of interest or emerging trends within auriculotherapy to guide their educational pursuits. Collaborating with other health professionals for multidisciplinary training can further broaden skill sets and treatment approaches. Sharing knowledge gained through continuing education with patients can foster trust and demonstrate a commitment to high-quality care.

Conclusion

Auriculotherapy offers a powerful and accessible method for pain relief, healing, and overall well-being. By understanding the key ear points, practicing safe techniques, and addressing common concerns, beginners can easily start their journey into ear acupuncture. Combining auriculotherapy with other therapies can enhance the healing process and provide holistic benefits. Whether you're a novice or looking to advance, ear acupuncture has great potential for promoting health naturally and effectively.

www.ingramcontent.com/pod-product-compliance
Lightning Source LLC
Chambersburg PA
CBHW071015250726
48653CB00005B/1625